Fast to Fit: The Ultimate Intermittent Fasting Handbook

Harness the Power of Fasting to Lose Weight, Boost Energy, Reduce Inflammation, and Feel Amazing

By: PRIYA MONICA

Copyright

© 2024 PRIYA MONICA. All rights reserved. No part of this publication may be reproduced, distributed, or transmitted in any form or by any means, including photocopying, recording, or other electronic or mechanical methods, without the prior written permission of the publisher, except in the case of brief quotations embodied in critical reviews and certain other noncommercial uses permitted by copyright law.

Disclaimer

The information presented in this book is for informational and educational purposes only. While the author has made every effort to ensure the accuracy and reliability of the information, it is not intended as a substitute for professional medical advice, diagnosis, or treatment. Always seek the advice of your physician or other qualified health provider with any questions you may have regarding a medical condition.

The use of recipes and supplements should be approached with care, and individuals should exercise caution and discretion when incorporating new remedies into their health regimen. The author and publisher are not liable for any adverse effects, injuries, or other consequences that may arise from using the information provided in this book.

These sections cover basic copyright protection and a standard disclaimer that protects you legally while clarifying that your book is not a substitute for professional medical advice. You can modify them according to your personal needs or legal requirements.

About the Author

Priya Monica is a passionate health and wellness advocate who believes in enabling others to live balanced, stress-free lives via mindful eating and holistic lifestyle choices. She is the author of several transformative books, including Carnivore Made Simple: A Beginner's Blueprint to Meat-Based Nutrition, The Keto Lifestyle for Beginners: Transform Your Health, Boost Energy, and Lose Weight for Life, and Cortisol Detox Diet Cookbook for Beginners, which focuses on stress management and hormone balance through nutritious recipes.

With a thorough grasp of the relationship between food and general well-being, Priya develops simple, science-backed recommendations to help readers adopt healthier lives. Her objective is to make health accessible to everyone, regardless of skill level or lifestyle restrictions. She thinks that taking focused, long-term measures may lead to revolutionary health results.

Priya's work includes practical instructions for speciality diets such as keto and carnivore, as well as tips for stress management and adrenal health. When she's not writing, she experiments with recipes, researches health trends, and offers her expertise via workshops and speaking engagements.

As an Indian author specializing in holistic treatment, Priya contributes her knowledge to works such as Diverticulitis Tea for Digestive Treatment and Diverticulitis Cookbook for Digestive Healing. Her work encourages readers to seek out natural, sustainable ways to well-being, stressing the healing power of food and lifestyle choices.

Stay connected with Priya Monica to learn about her newest publications, health suggestions, and more.

Table of Content

Copyright
Disclaimer
About the Author
Table of Content

Introduction
What is Intermittent Fasting?
Why Intermittent Fasting Works
Benefits of Reading This Book
Who This Book Is For
What to Expect From This Book

Chapter One:
Understanding Intermittent Fasting
The Science of Intermittent Fasting
Federal State vs. Fasting State
Autophagy
Hormonal Changes
How Fasting Affects Your Body
Key advantages of intermittent fasting
Common Myths and Misconceptions

Chapter Two:
Types of Intermittent Fasting Methods
1. The 16:8 Method (Time-Restricted Eating)
2. The 5:2 Method (The Fast Diet)
3. OMAD (One Meal a Day)
4. Alternate-Day Fasting (ADF)

5. 24-Hour Fasting (Eat-Stop-Eat)
6. The Warrior Diet
Choosing the Right Method for You

Chapter 3
Preparing for Intermittent Fasting
1. Mindset and Setting Realistic Goals
2) Gradual Transition: Begin softly and gradually build up.
3. Plan your meals and eat nutrient-dense foods.
4. Managing Hunger and adjusting to Fasting
5. Identifying and Overcoming Common Challenges.
Common obstacles and ways to overcome them:
6. The Importance Of Sleep And Stress Management
7. Maintaining Consistency and Evaluating Your Progress

Chapter 4:
Optimizing Your Intermittent Fasting Results
1. Combining Intermittent Fasting and Exercise
When to Exercise While Intermittent Fasting:
2. Nutritional Considerations to Maximize Results
What to Avoid When Eating Windows:
3. Maintaining Your Hormonal Health
Tips for maintaining hormonal health during fasting:
5. Overcoming plateaus and sustaining motivation

Chapter 5:
Tracking Your Results and Adjusting Your Plan
The Value of Tracking Your Results
Chapter 6:

Maintaining Long-Term Success with Intermittent Fasting
Key to Long-Term Success: Consistency and Flexibility
How to make fasting enjoyable
Integrating Intermittent Fasting with Other Health Practices.

Chapter 7:
Frequently Asked Questions About Intermittent Fasting
What is intermittent fasting and how does it work?
Can I drink water throughout my fasting period?
Other beverages to avoid when fasting:
Can I Take Supplements when Fasting?
Can I Exercise when fasting?
How Do I Know Whether I'm Eating Too Much or Too Little During My Eating Window?
What Happens If I Break My Fast By Accident?
How to Recover After Breaking Your Fast
Is intermittent fasting safe for everyone?
Can I Fast for a Longer period?
Will Intermittent Fasting Make Me Lose Muscle Mass?
Tips for preserving muscle mass when fasting:
How Do I Know If Intermittent Fasting Works for Me?
What happens if I stop intermittent fasting?

Chapter 8:
The Science Behind Intermittent Fasting
Mental Clarity and Brain Health.
How Fasting Improves Brain Health:
Longevity and ageing
How Fasting Affects Aging
Chapter 9:

Common Mistakes to Avoid While Fasting
Not staying hydrated.

Chapter 10:
Factors to Consider When Choosing a Fasting Schedule
How to Begin Your Fasting Plan
Sample Fasting Schedules

Chapter 11:
Overcoming Common Challenges While Fasting

Conclusion:
Your New Lifestyle – Making Fasting a Lifelong Habit

Bonus Section: Your Ultimate Guide to Fasting Success
Sample 7-Day Intermittent Fasting Plan
Meal Prep Ideas for Eating Windows

Introduction
What is Intermittent Fasting?

Intermittent fasting (IF) is an eating practice that alternates between fasting and eating. It focuses on when you eat rather than what you eat, allowing your body to automatically enter a fasting state at specified times throughout the day. This strategy might involve a variety of fasting windows, such as fasting for 16 hours and eating within an 8-hour window (known as the 16:8 method), fasting every other day, or fasting for 24 hours once or twice a week.

Intermittent fasting allows your body to metabolize food and burn fat for energy by limiting your meal times. It's simple to include in your daily routine, doesn't require any special meals or supplements, and has the potential to significantly improve your health. Unlike typical diets, which require continual calorie tracking or meal preparation, IF is adaptable to your lifestyle.

Why Intermittent Fasting Works

Intermittent fasting works by tapping into your body's natural cycles, allowing it to perform to its full capacity.

When you fast, your body goes through numerous crucial processes that help you lose weight, increase energy, and enhance your overall health.

First, fasting permits your body to switch to fat-burning mode. When you fast, insulin levels fall and your body shifts from burning glucose to burning stored fat. This process is referred to as ketosis. Furthermore, fasting activates autophagy, a process in which your body eliminates damaged cells and initiates cellular repair and regeneration, thus improving general health and lifespan.

While intermittent fasting does not necessitate a drastic change in diet, it does help balance hormones, reduce inflammation, and promote a consistent, continuous flow of energy throughout the day. This makes it a useful tool not only for weight reduction, but also for mental clarity, greater attention, and long-term health.

Benefits of Reading This Book

This book is intended to help you understand and apply intermittent fasting in a way that is appropriate for your lifestyle. You'll discover clear, actionable guidance on how to begin your fasting adventure, choose the best approach, and overcome frequent obstacles. This book provides a comprehensive overview of intermittent fasting and equips readers with strategies to efficiently lose weight using time-based eating patterns rather than restrictive diets. This kind of fasting will:

- Increase your energy levels and increase your mental sharpness.
- Improve your health by reducing inflammation, increasing metabolism, and controlling blood sugar levels.
- Feel great when you adopt a flexible dietary regimen that works into your hectic schedule.

Whether you're new to fasting or have tried it previously, this book will walk you through the basics, present tactics for sticking to it, and ensure you reap the full benefits of intermittent fasting without feeling overwhelmed.

Who This Book Is For

This book is intended for everyone who wants to learn more about the benefits of intermittent fasting for their health and body. This guide is designed for your specific goals, whether you want to lose weight, enhance your energy, reduce inflammation, or simply improve your general well-being.

If you're new to fasting, this book will take you through the science and show you how to get started safely and successfully. If you've attempted fasting before but struggled with consistency, this book can help you overcome typical problems and stay on track. If you're a busy professional, a student, a parent, or simply looking for a long-term strategy to enhance your lifestyle, you'll find tactics that fit around your schedule rather than against it.

What to Expect From This Book

This is more than just another diet book. It is a thorough handbook that combines the science of intermittent fasting with practical, easy-to-implement guidance. You'll learn about various fasting approaches, how to create attainable objectives, and how to incorporate fasting into your everyday routine. Along with practical counsel, you'll learn how to fuel your body with nutrient-dense meals, stay motivated, and conquer any challenges that emerge.

Each chapter is meant to provide you with the information you need to succeed, whether you're new to fasting or want to improve your practice. By the conclusion of this book, you'll not just understand how intermittent fasting works, but also how to make it work for you.

Chapter One:

Understanding Intermittent Fasting

Intermittent fasting (IF) is more than a fad; it's a strong, scientifically proven approach to improve your health and lose weight for good. However, to properly appreciate its advantages, we must first understand how and why fasting works. In this chapter, we'll look at the science underlying intermittent fasting, the physiological changes that occur during a fast, and the major advantages that make it such a powerful tool for health and weight control.

The Science of Intermittent Fasting

Intermittent fasting is fundamentally based on time. It focuses on when you eat, not what you consume. When you fast, your body switches from utilizing food as its major fuel source to burning stored fat. This procedure has been clinically demonstrated to aid with fat loss, metabolism, and cell repair. This is how it works.

Federal State vs. Fasting State

After eating, your body enters a fed state, in which it concentrates on digesting and processing the meal you just ate. The primary source of energy for your body is glucose (derived from carbs).

When you stop eating and enter a fasting state, insulin levels drop and your body starts to depend on stored fat for fuel. This is the condition in which fat is burned. During a fast, your body's metabolic processes change from breaking down food to breaking down fat cells, known as lipolysis.

Autophagy

One of the most interesting advantages of intermittent fasting is its capacity to stimulate autophagy, the body's natural process of removing damaged cells. Autophagy helps to eliminate damaged or defective proteins and cells, lowering the risk of a variety of illnesses such as cancer and neurological disorders.

Fasting triggers autophagy because your body knows that it is not receiving new nutrients and hence relies on existing resources to clean up and rebuild.

Hormonal Changes

Fasting causes numerous significant hormonal changes that promote weight reduction and overall wellness.

- Insulin: Following a meal, insulin levels increase to aid in the storage of nutrients. When you fast, insulin levels decrease, causing the body to burn fat.

- HGH (Human Growth Hormone) Fasting raises HGH levels, which aid in weight reduction, muscle retention, and general wellness.

- Ghrelin and Leptin: Fasting affects both ghrelin (which drives appetite) and leptin (which indicates fullness). Fasting gradually regulates these hormones, lowering appetite and making calorie management simpler.

How Fasting Affects Your Body

Fasting is an effective way to improve different elements of your health. Here are some of the major ways it helps your body:

- **Fat Loss and Weight Management**

One of the most evident and desired advantages of fasting is weight reduction. Fasting helps you lose fat by allowing your body more time to burn it rather than store it. In contrast to standard calorie-restricted diets, which may result in muscle loss, studies demonstrate that intermittent fasting is helpful for both fat reduction and retaining lean muscle mass.

- **Improved energy and mental clarity.**

Fasting helps to normalize blood sugar levels, avoiding the spikes and crashes that may make you feel lethargic. As a consequence, many individuals report having consistent energy levels throughout the day. Fasting induces ketosis, which has been related to improved mental clarity and attention. This is because ketones, an alternate fuel to glucose, are a very efficient energy source for the brain.

- **Improved Metabolism**

Fasting increases metabolic flexibility, which means your body may alternate between utilizing carbs and fat for energy based on availability. This capacity to burn fat as fuel might enhance insulin sensitivity, making it simpler to control blood sugar levels.

- **Reduced inflammation.**

Chronic inflammation is the underlying cause of several illnesses, including heart disease, diabetes, and cancer. According to research, intermittent fasting decreases inflammatory indicators in the body, possibly lessening the chance of developing certain illnesses.

- **Improved longevity**

Studies have indicated that fasting may activate genes linked to lifespan and illness prevention. Reduced inflammation, better metabolism, and autophagy all help you live longer, healthier lives.

Key advantages of intermittent fasting

In addition to the physical health benefits stated above, intermittent fasting has various lifestyle benefits that make it an appealing alternative for many people:

- **Simplicity and flexibility.**

Unlike standard diets that need intricate meal planning or calorie tracking, intermittent fasting is straightforward and adaptable. You do not need to substantially alter what you eat, but rather when you eat. This makes it simple to include in your routine.

- **Better mental health.**

There is evidence that intermittent fasting might boost mood and decrease anxiety. Fasting is thought to increase the release of brain-derived neurotrophic factor (BDNF), a protein that promotes brain health and cognitive performance.

- **Sustainable Lifestyle Change**

Unlike restrictive diets, which are difficult to stick to over time, intermittent fasting is a lifestyle modification that may be maintained continuously. Once you've become used to a fasting schedule, it becomes second nature and doesn't need continual attention or preparation.

Common Myths and Misconceptions

Despite its growing popularity, there are still many myths about intermittent fasting that can create confusion. Let's debunk some of the most common ones:

- **"Fasting Causes Starvation and Muscle Loss"**

Intermittent fasting preserves muscle mass, especially when combined with resistance training and adequate protein intake. It's important to note that fasting doesn't mean you're starving—it simply allows your body to access its fat stores for energy.

- "Fasting is Dangerous and Can Lead to Nutrient Deficiencies"

Intermittent fasting, when done correctly, is safe for most people and can improve nutrient absorption. It's crucial to eat nutrient-dense meals during your eating windows to ensure you're getting the vitamins and minerals your body needs.

- "You Have to Fast for Long Periods to See Results"

Many people assume that fasting for days at a time is necessary, but that's not true. Even shorter fasts—such as 16 hours of fasting and 8 hours of eating—can produce significant health benefits without requiring extreme or lengthy fasting periods.

- "Fasting Will Slow Down Your Metabolism"

Studies show that intermittent fasting can be abolished by increasing levels of norepinephrine, a hormone that helps burn fat. This is in contrast to calorie-restricted diets, which can often lead to a slowdown in metabolism.

Chapter Two:
Types of Intermittent Fasting Methods

There is no one-size-fits-all solution for intermittent fasting. Different techniques are appropriate for various situations, interests, and goals. The beauty of intermittent fasting is its adaptability—whether you want to lose weight, gain energy, or just improve your health, you may pick the fasting method that best meets your needs. In this chapter, we'll look at the most prevalent intermittent fasting tactics, their benefits, and how to pick which one is right for you.

1. The 16:8 Method (Time-Restricted Eating)

The 16:8 approach is one of the most popular and easy to use. It includes fasting for 16 hours and eating just within an 8-hour window each day. For example, you may choose to eat between 12:00 PM and 8:00 PM, skipping breakfast but eating lunch and dinner at that period.

How it works:

- You fast for 16 hours, which helps your body burn fat.

- You consume your daily calories in the remaining 8 hours, allowing you to have two or three meals.

Benefits:

- The 16:8 approach is straightforward to use, needing neither complex meal planning nor drastic nutritional changes.

- Flexibility: You may adjust the 8 hours to fit your schedule (10 AM to 6 PM, 12 PM to 8 PM).

- Consistency: Because it seamlessly integrates into most daily routines, 16:8 is easy to adopt as a lifelong habit.

Best for: Beginners and those looking for a manageable, sustainable approach to intermittent fasting.

2. The 5:2 Method (The Fast Diet)

Dr. Michael Mosley's 5:2 technique involves eating regularly five days a week and drastically reducing calories (about 500-600 calories) on the other two days. These fasting days are often spread apart, such as on Mondays and Thursdays.

How it works:

- For five days, eat consistently.
- On the other two days, you consume just 500-600 calories, which are often divided between several small meals.

Benefits:

- Flexibility: You just need to restrict your calories two days a week, giving enough room to eat normally the rest of the time.

- Simplicity: It's easy to follow since it's just about cutting calories on particular days, rather than continually fasting.

- Weight Loss: This method is popular with folks who want to shed weight and enhance their metabolic health.

Best for: Those who want to reduce calorie intake without having to fast daily or deal with long fasting periods.

3. OMAD (One Meal a Day)

The OMAD approach entails fasting for 23 hours each day and having one huge meal during the remaining 1-hour interval. It's an extreme kind of intermittent fasting, yet it can be quite successful for fat reduction and calorie restriction.

How it works:

- You consume a single substantial meal that is nutrition-rich and has all of the calories, protein, and vitamins you need for the day.
- You fast for the next 23 hours, drinking just water, herbal tea, or black coffee.

Benefits:

- Drastic Fat Loss: Limiting your eating window to just one meal makes it much simpler to create a calorie deficit, which promotes fat loss.

- Mental Clarity: Because of the lengthier fasting periods, many individuals report feeling more focused and clear-minded.

- Simplicity: You only have to worry about one meal every day, which makes meal preparation and planning easier.

Best for: Advanced fasters those seeking rapid weight loss, and individuals with busy schedules who don't want to spend time thinking about food throughout the day.

4. Alternate-Day Fasting (ADF)

As the name implies, alternate-day fasting entails switching between fasting and non-fasting days. On fasting days, you either eat nothing at all or limit your calories to about 500-600.

How it works:

- You alternate fasting and eating days. On eating days, you may eat regularly.
- On fasting days, you may either fast totally or eat a small quantity of food, depending on your preferences.

Benefits:

- Increased Fat Loss: This approach causes a high-calorie deficit over time, resulting in rapid fat loss.

- Cellular Repair: Extended fasting periods stimulate autophagy, which promotes cell repair and rejuvenation.

- Metabolic Flexibility: Intermittent fasting and eating improves metabolic health by improving insulin sensitivity.

Best for: Those who are experienced with fasting and are looking for a more intensive approach to fat loss.

5. 24-Hour Fasting (Eat-Stop-Eat)

The 24-hour fast entails fasting for 24 hours once or twice every week. For example, you may eat supper at 7:00 PM and then not eat again until 7:00 PM the following day. During the fasting time, you may have water, herbal tea, or black coffee but not solid foods.

How it works:

- You consume your last meal at the appropriate time and fast for 24 hours.
- You may repeat this fasting cycle once or twice a week, depending on how your body reacts.

- The fasting phase allows your body plenty of time to burn fat and reach profound ketosis.

Benefits:

- Accelerated Fat Burning: After 24 hours of fasting, your body enters a deep fat-burning mode, quickly emptying glycogen reserves and burning fat.

- Autophagy: A 24-hour fast increases autophagy, allowing your body to cleanse and repair cells.

- Improved Insulin Sensitivity: This approach reduces insulin resistance, resulting in improved blood sugar management.

Best for: Advanced fasters and individuals who want to push their fasting boundaries for quicker results.

6. The Warrior Diet

The Warrior Diet is built on the idea of eating little portions of fresh fruits and vegetables throughout the day and one huge meal at night. The eating window is usually approximately 4 hours, while the fasting phase lasts 20 hours.

How it works:

- You consume small portions of raw, natural foods (like fruits, vegetables, and juices) during the day to sustain energy levels.
- In the evening, you eat a large, well-balanced meal with plenty of protein, vegetables, and healthy fats.

Benefits:

- **Flexibility**: The Warrior Diet is a great way to incorporate fasting with clean eating without depriving yourself of essential nutrients during the day.
- **Effective Fat Loss**: Due to the long fasting period, the body remains fat-burning.
- **Detoxification**: The diet encourages cleansing the body with raw, unprocessed foods and plenty of hydration.

Best for: Those who prefer eating larger meals but want to maintain a fast for health benefits.

Choosing the Right Method for You

Which approach is ideal for you depends on your lifestyle, health objectives, and personal preferences. Here are some suggestions to help you decide:

- If you are a newbie, begin with the 16:8 approach. It's the most convenient and simple to include in your everyday routine.

- If you have a hectic schedule and want less frequent fasting, consider the 5:2 technique.

- Consider more sophisticated ways of fat reduction and health advantages, such as OMAD or Alternate-Day Fasting.

- If you want to experience profound cellular healing and detoxification, 24-hour fasting or the Warrior Diet may be an excellent option.

Remember that one approach is "better" than another; it all comes down to what works best for you and your objectives. As you continue reading, you'll discover how to efficiently incorporate these tactics into your daily routine and alter them as required for long-term success.

Chapter 3

Preparing for Intermittent Fasting

Starting an intermittent fasting diet may be life-changing for your health, but it requires cautious preparation. Fasting is more than just not eating; it's about understanding your body's needs, making adjustments, and setting yourself up for success. In this chapter, we'll look at the important components of preparing for intermittent fasting, such as mindset changes, meal planning, and coping with potential barriers.

1. Mindset and Setting Realistic Goals

Before going on an intermittent fasting journey, you must mentally prepare for success. Understanding why you want to fast and having measurable objectives will help you remain motivated and focused.

Steps for preparing your mindset:

- Understand Your "Why": Are you fasting to reduce weight, gain energy, enhance your metabolic health, or live longer? Knowing your "why" offers a greater sense of purpose and drive.
- Set reasonable expectations. Recognize that intermittent fasting is not a quick-fix diet. It is a progressive lifestyle change. You may experience initial hunger or weariness while your body

adapts, but these symptoms will pass. Be patient with yourself.
- Start slowly: If you're new to fasting, use an approach like 16:8 and gradually increase your fasting period. This allows your body to adapt without being overwhelmed.
- Track your progress: Keep a journal or use an app to track your eating patterns, hunger, energy levels, and other health metrics. Tracking can help you better understand how your body is responding and identify areas for improvement.

2) Gradual Transition: Begin softly and gradually build up.

One of the most frequent errors people make when beginning intermittent fasting is jumping in too soon. The body needs time to adjust to a new food pattern. Starting slowly decreases the possibility of overwhelming your system and raises the likelihood of long-term success.

How to ease into fasting:

- Ease Into Longer Fasts: If you're new to fasting, start with a shorter fasting window (like 12 hours) and gradually increase to 16 hours or more. For example, you may start by missing breakfast for a few days before gradually extending the fasting time.
- Adjust Your Having Window: If you're beginning with 16:8, try having your first meal later in the day to make fasting easier. For example, you may start eating at noon instead of 8:00 AM.
- Adjust as required. Listen to your body. If you feel extremely weary or furious during fasting, try shortening your fast or adjusting your meal times.

3. Plan your meals and eat nutrient-dense foods.

While intermittent fasting focuses on when you eat, the quality of your meals is as important. To make the most of your fast, fuel your body with nutrient-dense meals during your eating window. A well-balanced diet will keep you physically active, satisfy your hunger, and fuel your body, resulting in optimal health.

Tips for Meal Planning:

- Choose nutrient-dense whole foods like vegetables, lean meats, healthy fats (avocado, olive oil, nuts), and complex carbohydrates (whole grains, legumes). These will help to normalize your blood sugar levels and provide long-term energy.
- Avoid processed food. Consuming processed foods rich in sugar or refined carbs may produce blood sugar fluctuations, making fasting more challenging.
- Aim for a balanced macronutrient intake, which includes protein, fats, and carbohydrates. Protein is particularly important for muscle maintenance, while healthy fats increase satiety.
- Stay Hydrated: Drink plenty of water throughout the day, particularly during fasts. You may also drink herbal teas or black coffee, but sugary drinks will disturb you fast.
- Meal Times and Portions: During your eating window, try to have two or three balanced meals or one larger meal (if following OMAD). Portion

control is vital for avoiding overeating during your meal window.

4. Managing Hunger and adjusting to Fasting

Hunger may be one of the most challenging challenges when beginning intermittent fasting. However, when your body adjusts, your hunger levels will normalize, making fasting easier. Here are several ways to manage hunger during fasting periods:

Strategies for managing hunger:

- Drink Plenty of Water: Water not only hydrates but also regulates hunger. If you feel hungry when fasting, sip some water. Herbal teas and black coffee (without sugar or milk) are also great options.
- Stay busy: Distracting oneself with activities like as taking a stroll, working, or doing something enjoyable may help you forget about eating.
- Consume nutrient-dense meals. Make sure your meals inside your eating window are nutritionally dense. This will allow you to remain fuller for longer and prevent feeling hungry later.

- Adapt your meals: Eat extra fibre-rich foods like veggies, fruits, and whole grains to feel fuller longer. Protein and healthy fats are also necessary for remaining satiated.

5. Identifying and Overcoming Common Challenges.

Starting intermittent fasting may provide some challenges. To stay on track, it's vital to recognize these issues early on and understand how to solve them.

Common obstacles and ways to overcome them:

- Hunger pangs: At first, you may feel hungry, especially if you are accustomed to eating often. This is normal and will pass after your body adjusts. You may offset this by drinking water, sipping herbal tea, or doing anything else to distract yourself.
- Energy Slump: Some people feel tired or sluggish when they first begin fasting. If this happens, make sure you are obtaining enough nutrition during your meal period, especially protein and healthy fats. Once your body has adjusted, your energy levels should return to normal.

- Social Events and Meals Out: It may be difficult to maintain a fasting schedule when attending social events or eating out. Plan ahead of time by choosing fasting periods that work with your schedule or adjusting your fasting strategy for special occasions.
- Cravings: Sugar or junk food cravings may develop throughout the fasting period, especially in the beginning. The idea is to eat substantial, nutrient-dense meals that keep you satisfied. As your body adjusts to fasting, your cravings will gradually fade.

6. The Importance Of Sleep And Stress Management

While intermittent fasting is mostly about food and meal time, other areas of health, such as sleep and stress management, are also important for success. Poor sleep and excessive stress levels might impair your ability to fast properly and induce hormonal imbalances that affect your appetite and metabolism.

Tips for Improved Sleep and Stress Management:

- Prioritize Sleep: Aim for 7-9 hours of quality sleep every night. Poor sleep may cause cravings and alter hunger hormones, making fasting more difficult.

- Manage Stress: High-stress levels might cause emotional eating or increased hunger, making it harder to fast. Deep breathing, yoga, or meditation may all help you relax and manage stress.
- Exercise regularly: Include regular physical activity in your routine. Exercise may help you balance your hormones, reduce stress, and lose weight.

7. Maintaining Consistency and Evaluating Your Progress

As you begin your intermittent fasting adventure, consistency is essential. It's important to make changes as you go, be patient with the process, and celebrate minor triumphs along the way.

Ways to Stay On Track:

- Evaluate your progress: Keep note of your mood, weight, and energy levels, as well as how you're reacting to fasting. Consider taking measurements

and tracking your improvement in a notebook or app.
- Maintain flexibility. Life happens, and you may need to adjust your fasting schedule. That is okay! Be versatile and responsive to your changing needs.
- Celebrate Milestones: Celebrate your successes along the way. Whether you're losing weight, feeling more energetic, or just sticking to your fasting plan for a week, every victory is worth celebrating.

Chapter 4:
Optimizing Your Intermittent Fasting Results

Intermittent fasting may improve health, weight reduction, and general well-being. However, to fully reap the advantages of fasting, you need to apply a few tactics that will help you reach your objectives quicker and more efficiently. In this chapter, we will look at how to improve your intermittent fasting outcomes by combining it with exercise, diet, and other good lifestyle practices.

1. Combining Intermittent Fasting and Exercise

Exercise is an important part of a healthy lifestyle, and when combined with intermittent fasting, it may dramatically increase the benefits of both disciplines. Fasting, on the other hand, requires time and intensity.

Best exercises for intermittent fasting:

- Strength Training: Lifting weights or doing bodyweight workouts (push-ups, squats, lunges) may help you gain muscle mass, which enhances your metabolism and promotes fat reduction. Strength training is best done during your eating window when you have plenty of energy.
- Cardio: Aerobic workouts such as walking, running, cycling, or swimming might help you burn more fat, particularly if you fast beforehand.

Because your body uses fat as its major energy source, fasted exercise is great at targeting fat deposits.
- High-intensity interval training (HIIT): HIIT is a time-saving workout in which you alternate between short bursts of intensive exertion and rest. HIIT may be done while fasting, and it has been demonstrated to increase fat reduction and enhance cardiovascular health.

When to Exercise While Intermittent Fasting:

- Before breaking your fast: If you prefer cardio or high-intensity interval training, try exercising in the morning before your first meal. Fasting allows for greater fat oxidation and endurance.
- After Eating: If you're performing strength training, it's usually best to work out after your first meal or throughout your eating period. This ensures that you have enough fuel for muscle repair and development.

Considerations:

- Listen to your body: If you feel tired or lightheaded during an exercise, it might be

because you're not eating enough or your body needs more time to acclimate to fasting.
- Take a rest, drink, and alter your meal schedule as necessary.

2. Nutritional Considerations to Maximize Results

Intermittent fasting is not just about when you eat, but also about what you consume. Fueling your body with the correct nutrition throughout your eating windows will help you achieve your fasting goals and stay energized.

Important nutrients to prioritize:

- Protein is necessary for muscle repair, satiety, and maintaining lean body mass. Make sure each meal has a decent supply of protein, such as chicken, fish, tofu, lentils, or eggs.
- Healthy Fats: Fats help you stay full and promote overall wellness. Include healthy fats from avocados, olive oil, nuts, and seeds.
- Fibre-rich foods (vegetables, fruits, whole grains) promote digestive health and increase feelings of fullness. Eating a fibre-rich meal will assist in curbing appetite during fasting times.

- Micronutrients: Vitamins and minerals are essential for good health. To guarantee an appropriate spectrum of micronutrients, consume a variety of coloured vegetables and fruits.
- Hydration: Staying hydrated is essential for successful intermittent fasting. Water, herbal teas, and electrolytes may help you avoid dehydration, which can impair your fasting performance and make you feel lethargic.

What to Avoid When Eating Windows:

- Sugary, processed foods: These foods may raise your blood sugar levels, resulting in insulin resistance and appetite after eating. To maintain steady blood sugar levels, eat full, unprocessed meals.
- Excessive carbohydrates: While carbohydrates are necessary for energy, particularly after exercise, eating too many simple carbs might negate the advantages of intermittent fasting. Rather than processed sweets and white bread, choose

complex carbohydrates such as sweet potatoes, quinoa, or whole grains.

3. Maintaining Your Hormonal Health

Intermittent fasting has a significant influence on your hormones and, when done appropriately, may result in improved metabolic health, weight reduction, and overall well-being. Understanding the function of hormones in fasting might help you enhance your outcomes and prevent possible problems.

Intermittent fasting affects the following key hormones:

- Insulin: Intermittent fasting lowers insulin levels, which promotes fat loss. Lower insulin levels also aid in preventing the buildup of extra fat.
- Fasting promotes the release of growth hormone, which is essential for muscle gain, fat reduction, and cellular repair.
- Leptin is the hormone that regulates appetite and energy levels. As you lose fat, your body becomes

more sensitive to leptin, which makes you feel full and pleased.
- Cortisol: Cortisol, the stress hormone, may increase when fasting. While a certain amount of cortisol is acceptable, high quantities may cause exhaustion, irritation, and difficulties losing weight. To regulate cortisol production, minimize stress and get adequate sleep.

Tips for maintaining hormonal health during fasting:

- Avoid Over-Fasting: While fasting has hormonal advantages, fasting for extended periods without an appropriate diet may raise cortisol levels and impair thyroid function. Find the right balance for you.
- Manage Stress: Excessive stress may affect hormone balance and make fasting harder. Incorporate stress-relieving hobbies such as meditation, yoga, and deep breathing techniques into your daily routine.
- Prioritize Sleep: Adequate sleep is necessary for hormonal equilibrium. Aim for 7-9 hours of sleep every night to help your body heal, balance hormones, and recover from fasting and exercise.

4. Adjusting Your Fasting Schedule

One of the most important aspects of intermittent fasting is figuring out what fasting schedule works best for you. This may change based on your health objectives, daily schedule, and preferences. Fine-tuning your schedule can help you to get the most out of fasting without feeling deprived or stressed.

Ways to Change Your Fasting Schedule:

- Experiment with several methods: Try multiple fasting strategies (16:8, 5:2, OMAD) to find which one best fits your lifestyle and objectives. You may discover that a mix of fasting patterns works best for you.
- Modify Eating Windows: If you notice that your hunger peaks at specific times of the day, adapt your meal schedule appropriately. For example, if you are not hungry in the morning but desire food late at night, change your eating window to 12 - 8 p.m. or later.
- Include Refeeds and Breaks: To avoid metabolic slowdown and enhance long-term sustainability, some individuals prefer to take fasting breaks

every few weeks or cycle in higher-calorie days (known as refeed days).

5. Overcoming plateaus and sustaining motivation

It is usual to reach a plateau in weight reduction or health improvement while following an intermittent fasting routine. This might be disappointing, but remember that growth isn't always linear. Instead of giving up, use the following ways to overcome plateaus and stay motivated.

Tips for Overcoming Plateaus:

- Track your progress: Keep note of your measurements, weight, energy level, and other indicators of success. This will keep you motivated even if you don't notice instant progress on the scale.
- Increase exercise intensity: If you've been doing low-intensity activities, try adding more difficult exercises or extending your workout time. Resistance training and high-intensity exercises might help you break past a plateau.
- Adjust your fasting protocol: If you've been following the same fasting routine for a long, try something different. You may need to change

your eating schedule, cut calories on fasting days, or attempt a more complex strategy such as OMAD.
- Stay Consistent: Plateaus are often just transient states. Maintain consistency in your fasting, exercise, and dietary habits. The results will ultimately arrive.

<u>Maintaining Motivation:</u>

- Set milestones: Celebrate little victories, such as completing a certain amount of fasting hours or dropping a few pounds. These milestones will keep you motivated.
- Find a Support System: Share your experiences with a friend, family member, or online community. Having someone to chat with and share experiences with might help you stay motivated.
- Focus on Non-Scale Victories: Sometimes the greatest development is not evident on the scale. Concentrate on improving your energy, sleep quality, mood, and general wellness.

Chapter 5:

Tracking Your Results and Adjusting Your Plan

Tracking your progress is essential in any health journey, particularly with intermittent fasting. Whether you're attempting to lose weight, increase your energy, or reach other health goals, tracking your progress lets you identify what's working, what needs to be altered, and how to keep going. In this chapter, we'll look at how to effectively assess your intermittent fasting results, what metrics to monitor, and how to fine-tune your plan for long-term success.

The Value of Tracking Your Results

Intermittent fasting is a dynamic process that influences eating habits, metabolism, and body composition. Tracking is critical for knowing how well your fasting plan is working for you. Not only does it provide you with a clear picture of your progress, but it also keeps you accountable and motivated.

Why tracking matters:

- Evaluate efficacy. Regular monitoring helps you to assess if you are achieving the desired results, such as weight loss, more energy, or improved mental clarity.
- Identify adjustment areas: If you've hit a plateau or believe your progress has slowed, monitoring

may help you identify potential reasons, such as insufficient calorie intake, stress, or a lack of exercise.
- Maintain motivation: Seeing the results of your efforts may help you remain motivated, especially when you achieve goals like decreasing weight, building muscle, or feeling more energetic.

Key Metrics To Track

Tracking the right metrics ensures that you're tracking the aspects of your health and fasting journey that are important to your goals. Here are the most important metrics to look at.

1. Weight and physical measurements.

- Scale Weight: While weight is an obvious metric, it's important to realize that it doesn't tell the whole story. Weight fluctuations might occur due to water retention, muscular development, or other factors.
- Body Measurements: Take measurements of your waist, hips, arms, and thighs to track changes in body composition. Fat loss is often more noticeable in measurements than on the scale.

- Body fat percentage: If possible, use a body fat scale or calliper to monitor changes in body fat percentage. Losing fat, not weight is the ultimate goal in terms of health and body composition.

2. Energy levels.

Track your energy levels throughout the day. On a scale of 1 to 10, rate your energy levels when you get up, during lunch, and before going to bed. This can help you determine if fasting improves your overall energy or whether adjustments are needed.

3. Hunger and desires.

Keep note of how often and powerfully you feel hunger and desire while fasting. This may help you determine how well your body is responding to fasting and if you need to adjust your meal timings or food choices.

4. Sleep quality.

Sleep is essential for effective fasting. Monitor your sleep quality, amount, and duration. A good night's sleep is crucial for weight loss, vitality, and overall health.

5. Mental clarity and focus.

Throughout the day, keep track of your attention and mental focus. Some people believe that fasting helps them focus, while others experience brain fog. Monitor how fasting affects your mental clarity.

6. Exercise performance.

Keep track of your performance during the workouts. Do you lift more weights, run faster, or feel more energized when exercising? This may assist you assess if fasting helps or hinders your fitness growth.

7. Blood markers and health indicators.

If you want to be more exact, you may monitor your blood sugar, cholesterol levels, and other key health markers. Regular check-ups with a healthcare practitioner may help assess how intermittent fasting impacts your general health.

Tools for Tracking

You may monitor your findings using several tools and techniques, ranging from basic pen and paper to more modern technologies. Here are a few choices:

1. Journal & Log

- Food and Fasting Journal: Keep track of what and when you eat, as well as how you feel during fasting times. This is a fantastic way to monitor trends, identify problem areas, and ensure you stick to your fasting schedule.
- Exercise Journal: Track your workouts, including the kind, duration, intensity, and progress. This will allow you to assess the effectiveness of combining exercise with fasting.
- Mood and Energy Tracker: Keep track of your energy level, mood, and hunger. This will assist you in identifying trends and determining how your body is reacting to intermittent fasting.

2. Application and Technology:

- Apps like Zero, Fastient, and Life Fasting Tracker may help you record fasting hours, monitor progress, and get reminders to stay on track. They often include features like goal setting, trend tracking, and sharing your success with others.
- Fitness Tracking Apps: Apps like MyFitnessPal, Cronometer, and Fitbit may help you track your calories, macronutrients, exercise routines, and progress over time.

- Body Measuring Tools: Use a body fat scale or a smart scale to track your weight, body fat percentage, and muscle mass. These tools may allow you to get a more accurate picture of your body's composition over time.

3. Blood Tests and Health Monitoring

- Regular checkups: If possible, schedule frequent checkups with your doctor to monitor your blood sugar, cholesterol, thyroid function, and other key health markers. This may help you get a comprehensive understanding of how fasting impacts your overall health.
- Wearable Devices: Devices like the Oura Ring and Whoop Strap may measure sleep, heart rate variability, and other health indicators, offering additional information on how your body reacts to fasting.

4. Changing Your Fasting Plan Based On Results

After monitoring your results for a few weeks, it's time to assess your progress and make changes. This stage is necessary to continue progressing and overcome plateaus.

Here's how to modify your strategy depending on what you've tracked:

1. If weight loss is slow or stalled:

- Increase exercise intensity: If you've been doing largely gentle exercise, try including strength training or increasing the intensity of your routines.
- Reduce Caloric Intake: You may need to eat somewhat less during your meal window or change the sorts of foods you consume. To boost fat loss, eat more whole foods, high-protein meals, and healthy fats.
- Extend Fasting Hours: whether you're on a 16:8 fasting schedule, consider a longer fasting window (18:6 or 20:4) to see whether it speeds up fat loss.

2. Adjust Your Eating Window:

- If you feel tired or low on energy, try reducing your fast or eating more often. For some individuals, fasting for lengthy periods might cause weariness, so find a balance that works for you.
- Improve Your Sleep Quality: Make sure you receive adequate rest. Poor sleep may have an

impact on your energy levels, emotions, and metabolism.
- Check your Macronutrient Intake: Make sure you're getting enough protein and healthy fats to power your exercises and everyday activities.

3. **To manage hunger or cravings:**

- Prioritize fibre and protein. Increase the fibre and protein in your meals. These nutrients allow you to feel satiated for longer times.
- Drink More Water: Feeling hungry might be an indication of dehydration. Drink plenty of water throughout the day, and consider using herbal teas or electrolyte drinks during fasting times.
- Modify the Fasting Windows: If a 16:8 schedule does not work for you, consider a 14:10 or 12:12 strategy to gradually transition into longer fasting periods.

4. **If You're Not Getting the Mental Clarity You Want:**

- Consider Your Food Choices. Consume nutrient-dense foods that promote brain function, such as avocados, leafy greens, lean meats, and healthy fats (for example, omega-3s).

- Reduce Stress: High-stress levels might impair mental clarity. To clear your thoughts, try stress-relieving activities such as yoga, meditation, or deep breathing.
- Adjust Your Fast Duration: Some individuals have cognitive fog during prolonged fasts, while others flourish in a fasted condition. Try varying your fasting duration to see if it enhances your concentration.

5. Celebrating Your Progress

Tracking is more than simply finding areas for growth; it's also about recognizing your accomplishments. Every minor triumph, from a decrease in body fat percentage to increased energy levels, indicates that you are getting closer to your objectives. Recognize your success, whether it's reaching a weight goal, setting a new personal best in your exercises, or feeling more energy throughout the day.

How to Celebrate Your Progress:

- Reward yourself: After reaching a milestone, reward yourself with something unique, such as a massage, new training clothing, or a day off.
- Reflect on your journey: Take a look at your results and admire how far you've come.
- Write down all you've learnt from monitoring and how it's influenced your health journey.

Chapter 6:
Maintaining Long-Term Success with Intermittent Fasting

Intermittent fasting may be a very successful technique for weight reduction, health improvement, and increased energy. However, the true issue frequently arises when it comes to maintaining such outcomes over time. Fasting is not a fast cure; it is a lifestyle change that must be incorporated into your daily routine to ensure long-term success. In this chapter, we'll look at ways to reap the long-term advantages of intermittent fasting while also making it a sustainable and fun part of your lifestyle.

Key to Long-Term Success: Consistency and Flexibility

While consistency is essential for intermittent fasting, flexibility is also vital. Life happens—there will be social gatherings, holidays, or times when adhering to a rigorous fasting regimen is impossible. The key to long-term success is understanding how to tailor your fasting schedule to your lifestyle while being dedicated to your overall health objectives.

Why consistency matters:

- Keeping to the routine: When you continuously adhere to your intermittent fasting plan, your body adjusts to your eating habits, making it simpler to regulate hunger and sustain energy levels.
- Developing habits: Fasting becomes second nature over time when practised regularly. This makes fasting a habit, lowering mental effort and increasing long-term adherence.

Why flexibility matters:

- Life's events and memorable occasions: Being excessively strict about your fasting regimen might cause extra stress, particularly when attending social gatherings or during the holidays. Allowing oneself some freedom will keep fasting from feeling like a hardship.
- Adjusting your schedule: If your routine changes due to job, family, or other obligations, modify your fasting schedule to accommodate your new lifestyle. Shortening or extending your fasting windows as needed guarantees that you may continue fasting without feeling constrained.

How to make fasting enjoyable

To continue intermittent fasting as a lifestyle, it must be fun. If you detest your fasting schedule or feel starved, you're more inclined to skip it. There are easy methods to turn fasting into a rewarding and helpful part of your day.

1. Increase Variety in Your Meals:

- Flavorful and nutrient-dense foods: When you break your fast, be sure to include tasty, whole-food meals that will keep you full and eager to eat. Experiment with various cuisines and cooking methods to keep your meals interesting and new.
- Try different recipes: Cooking may provide a creative outlet. To keep meals interesting, try new foods, various herbs and spices, and taste combinations.

2. Social Support:

- Find a fasting friend. Having a friend or family member who observes intermittent fasting will help you stay motivated. You may discuss your experiences, brainstorm meal ideas, and keep each other responsible.

- Join online communities. Many online communities and forums concentrate on intermittent fasting. These forums allow you to share your experiences, ask questions, and learn from others.

3. Treat Yourself Occasionally:

Enjoy the odd treat: While it is vital to eat healthily most of the time, giving yourself occasional pleasures may help reduce feelings of deprivation and make fasting more lasting. Balance is essential for every special occasion, whether it's a holiday dinner or a favourite delicacy at a party.

The Impact of Mindset on Long-Term Success

Maintaining a good mentality is key to long-term success with intermittent fasting. How you think about fasting will determine how devoted you are to the practice. A healthy, empowered mentality may help you convert obstacles into chances for development and stay motivated even when progress seems sluggish.

1. Transition from a "diet" to a "lifestyle" perspective.

- Fasting should not be seen as a quick remedy. Many individuals struggle with dieting because they believe it produces only momentary effects. Change your perspective to see intermittent fasting as a lifetime commitment to health and fitness. When you accept fasting as a sustainable lifestyle, you are less inclined to return to previous behaviours.
- Be patient with your body. Remember that progress takes time, and it's common to have plateaus or setbacks. Instead of concentrating just on the scale, be patient and consider how fasting might help your health.

2. Overcome negative ideas.

- Combat hunger with optimistic thoughts: It's natural to feel hungry when fasting, but instead of concentrating on the pain, remember why you're fasting. Consider the health advantages you're receiving and how fasting corresponds with your long-term objectives.
- Celebrate minor successes. Celebrate every achievement, no matter how minor. Recognize your accomplishments, whether it's more energy,

better sleep, or weight loss, to maintain a good outlook.

Dealing With Challenges Over Time

As you continue with intermittent fasting, you may encounter problems such as social gatherings, emotional eating, or a hectic schedule. These challenges might throw off your fasting pattern, but with the correct tactics, they can be handled.

1. Fasting on social occasions:

- Plan ahead of time: If you know there will be an occasion where you will be tempted to eat outside of your typical window, base your fasting schedule on that. If necessary, adjust your eating schedule to meet the function, or eat light before the gathering and enjoy the social component without feeling obligated to eat.
- Maintain focus on your goals: While it is OK to indulge during social occasions, always remind yourself of why you are fasting. Choose to enjoy yourself without feeling bad about your eating choices.

2. Emotional Eating:

- Identify stressors that might disrupt your fasting strategy. Take note of any emotional triggers (stress, boredom, or melancholy) that cause you to eat outside of your fasting period. To control these feelings, try practices such as writing, mindfulness, or deep breathing.
- Find alternatives. Prepare a strategy for dealing with emotional desires. Take a stroll, sip herbal tea, or participate in an enjoyable activity to divert your attention away from eating and cope with emotions healthfully.

3. Travel and busy schedules:

- Be adaptive. Travelling or having a busy schedule does not require you to stop your fasting regimen. Pack nutritious snacks or meals that fall inside your eating window, and attempt to maintain consistency even when on the road.
- Embrace flexibility: Your fasting schedule may not always be ideal when travelling. It's critical to be adaptable and modify as required. Don't worry about a day or two of unsatisfactory fasting; simply get back on track as quickly as possible.

Integrating Intermittent Fasting with Other Health Practices.

Intermittent fasting works best when accompanied by other healthy habits like exercise, stress management, and proper sleep hygiene. These behaviours complement and increase fasting's effects. Here's how you can combine fasting with other lifestyle habits:

1. Exercise regularly:

- Find a regimen that works for you. Incorporate cardio and strength training into your program to boost fat reduction, muscle gain, and overall fitness. Exercise not only complements but also enhances the advantages of fasting, such as increased metabolism and hormonal balance.
- Exercise during the fasting window: Many individuals find that exercising during fasting times promotes fat burning and energy levels.

2. Managing Stress:

- Practice mindfulness. Integrating mindfulness activities such as meditation or deep breathing into your daily routine might help reduce cortisol levels, making fasting simpler and less stressful.

- Engage in soothing activities: Stress may impair your ability to keep to a fast, so choose things that soothe you, such as yoga, reading, or spending time outside.

3. Prioritize Sleep:

Ensure adequate sleep. Sleep is crucial for healing, metabolism, and general health. Aim for 7-9 hours of peaceful sleep every night to aid in your body's recovery after fasting and activity. Poor sleep may slow weight reduction and disrupt hunger hormones, making fasting more difficult to continue.

Chapter 7:
Frequently Asked Questions About Intermittent Fasting

Intermittent fasting is becoming more popular as a health practice, but it also raises numerous problems. Whether you are new to fasting or have been practising for a long, you may have questions or concerns. In this chapter, we'll answer the most commonly asked questions regarding intermittent fasting, aiming to clear up any misconceptions and provide you with the knowledge you need to succeed on your fasting journey.

What is intermittent fasting and how does it work?

Intermittent fasting is an eating pattern in which you alternate between periods of eating and fasting. Unlike typical diets, which concentrate on what you eat, intermittent fasting is more concerned with when you eat. Fasting is thought to help your body burn fat more effectively, enhance metabolism, and promote general health by giving your body a break from processing meals.

How It Works: During fasting, your body enters a state of ketosis, in which it switches from burning glucose (food) to burning fat for energy. This may result in weight reduction, enhanced metabolic health, and even greater mental clarity.

Can I drink water throughout my fasting period?

Yes! Staying hydrated during fasting times is critical to your health. Water, herbal teas, and black coffee are all excellent choices that will not disrupt your fast. In reality, drinking enough water reduces appetite, aids digestion, and keeps your body running smoothly.

Other beverages to avoid when fasting:

- Sugar-sweetened drinks: These will break your fast and cause an increase in insulin levels.
- Milk: Even small amounts of milk include calories and sugar, which may disrupt the fasting process.

Can I Take Supplements when Fasting?

- Yes, most supplements will not break your fast if they are free of calories and sweets. However, there are several factors to consider:
- Electrolytes: If you're fasting for a long time, you may need to restore your electrolytes (sodium,

potassium, and magnesium) since fasting may produce imbalances.
- Vitamins: Fat-soluble vitamins (A, D, E, and K) are best taken with meals since they need fat to absorb. They may be consumed with your first meal after fasting, but be careful if taken on an empty stomach.
- Always check the label and ensure that your supplements include no additional sweets or calories.

Can I Exercise when fasting?

Yes, you may exercise while fasting, but how you feel will be determined by the intensity of the activity and your body's adaptation to fasting. Many individuals find that low- to moderate-intensity exercises, such as walking or yoga, are acceptable during fasting times. Others may prefer higher-intensity exercises after they've adjusted to the fasting schedule.

Tips for Exercise when Fasting:

- Begin with low-impact workouts to let your body acclimate.
- Drink a lot of water before and after exercising.

- If you feel lightheaded or weak after fasting for a lengthy period, avoid exercising.
- If you're undertaking high-intensity exercises, you may want to break your fast with a little meal to replenish your energy.

How Do I Know Whether I'm Eating Too Much or Too Little During My Eating Window?

When practising intermittent fasting, it is important to pay attention to your body. There is no need to overeat during your eating window, but you should consume enough calories and minerals to power your body and maintain your health.

Signs You're Eating Too Much:

- Following meals, you may feel too full or unpleasant.
- Despite having regular fasting times, I'm gaining weight.
- Feeling slow or lethargic after eating.
- Signs You're Eating Too Little:
- Continuous hunger or urges during fasting times.
- Low energy or tiredness.
- Difficulty concentrating.

Finding Balance:

Aim for nutrient-dense meals that include healthy fats, proteins, and fibre. These meals can help you stay fuller for longer and maintain consistent energy levels. Pay attention to your hunger signals and eat until you're satisfied, not full.

What Happens If I Break My Fast By Accident?

Do not worry! If you mistakenly eat or drink anything during a fasting time, just resume your fasting at the next available opportunity. Fasting is a flexible discipline, so one slip-up will not derail your progress. The idea is to maintain consistency throughout time.

How to Recover After Breaking Your Fast

- Accept what occurred and avoid feeling guilty.
- Continue fasting as scheduled.
- Concentrate on being devoted to your overall objectives.
- Learn from the experience and determine what caused the error so that it does not happen again.

Is intermittent fasting safe for everyone?

Intermittent fasting is typically considered safe for most healthy people. However, some populations should see a healthcare practitioner before initiating an intermittent fasting routine, including:

- Pregnant and nursing women: Fasting may not be acceptable during pregnancy or nursing due to increased nutritional demands.
- People with eating disorders: Those with a history of eating problems may discover that fasting leads to poor eating habits.
- People with specific medical conditions: If you have diabetes, hypoglycemia, or any other chronic illness, you should see your doctor before beginning intermittent fasting.
- If you have any concerns about intermittent fasting, you should consult with a healthcare physician first.

Can I Fast for a Longer period?

While intermittent fasting normally consists of fasting for 12-24 hours, some individuals engage in longer fasting (greater than 24 hours) for unique health advantages. Extended fasting should be approached with caution, and it is critical to contact a healthcare practitioner before trying lengthier fasts.

Risks of Extended Fasting:

- Dehydration
- Electrolyte imbalances
- Nutritional deficiencies
- Loss of muscular mass

If you're new to fasting, start with shorter fasts (12-16 hours) and gradually work your way up to longer fasting periods as your body adjusts.

Will Intermittent Fasting Make Me Lose Muscle Mass?

Intermittent fasting is unlikely to induce muscle loss if you consume enough protein and engage in regular strength training workouts. In reality, fasting may assist in maintaining muscle mass while accelerating fat reduction by increasing insulin and growth hormone production efficiency.

Tips for preserving muscle mass when fasting:

- Strength Training: Incorporate weightlifting or bodyweight workouts into your workout.
- Adequate protein intake: Make sure your meals are high in protein to aid with muscle repair and development.
- Consume nutrient-rich meals: To promote general health, eat entire, nutrient-dense meals.

How Do I Know If Intermittent Fasting Works for Me?

Intermittent fasting is effective when you see changes in your weight, energy, mental clarity, and general health. Common indicators that fasting is effective include:

- Weight loss (fat loss, not just water weight)
- Increased energy levels throughout the day
- Better digestion, less bloating.
- Increased mental clarity and concentration
- Improved sleep quality.

Remember that the procedure takes time. To assess improvement, be patient and document your outcomes continuously.

What happens if I stop intermittent fasting?

When you end intermittent fasting, you may notice various changes in your body. These changes are often connected to how your body processes food and expends energy. If you return to eating frequent meals and snacks, you may gain weight, have a slower metabolism, and have fluctuating energy levels.

It is crucial to highlight, however, that intermittent fasting should never be seen as a "quick fix" but rather as a long-term strategy for health. If you quit fasting, you may still get many of the advantages of following a nutritious diet and exercising regularly.

Chapter 8:

The Science Behind Intermittent Fasting

Intermittent fasting is more than a fad; it has scientific roots. Understanding the physiological mechanisms that occur while fasting might help you understand the health advantages while also making the practice more successful. In this chapter, we will look at the science behind intermittent fasting, including how it impacts your metabolism, hormones, and cells. With a greater knowledge of these systems, you will be able to utilize fasting as a tool to improve your health.

Metabolic Shift: From Glucose to Fat Burning.

One of the key advantages of intermittent fasting is that it allows your body to change its primary fuel source from glucose (sugar) to fat. This shift happens when your glycogen reserves, the body's stored form of glucose, are depleted, and your body begins to burn fat for energy.

How It Works:

- Glycemic depletion: During the fasting phase, your body depletes its glycogen reserves from the liver and muscles. When these stockpiles are

exhausted (typically after 12-16 hours of fasting), your body uses fat as its next fuel source.
- Fat Burning: As your body begins to burn fat for fuel, it enters a stage known as lipolysis, in which stored fat is broken down into fatty acids and glycerol that may be utilized as energy.
- Ketosis: If you continue to fast, your body may enter a condition called ketosis, in which fat is turned into ketones. These ketones provide an alternate fuel source for the brain and body.

This metabolic shift is responsible for the majority of the fat loss that happens during intermittent fasting. It also improves insulin sensitivity, which may lower the risk of metabolic illnesses such as type 2 diabetes.

Hormonal Changes for Weight Loss

Fasting causes several hormonal reactions that promote weight reduction and general wellness. Intermittent fasting affects the following important hormones:

1. What Insulin Does: Insulin is a hormone produced by the pancreas in reaction to meals, specifically carbs. It helps to control blood sugar levels by letting cells absorb glucose from the circulation.

Fasting impact: When you fast, your insulin levels decrease considerably, allowing your body to burn fat more efficiently. Lower insulin levels also aid in fat accumulation because insulin blocks the release of fat from fat cells.

2. HGH: What It Does: Human growth hormone promotes muscular development, fat reduction, and general cellular repair.

Fasting has a positive influence on HGH levels, which helps to preserve muscle mass while losing weight and accelerates fat burning. Fasting may boost HGH levels by up to five times.

3. Ghrelin (The Hunger Hormone): Ghrelin promotes hunger and signals the brain when it's time to eat.

Fasting impact: Ghrelin levels normally increase during fasting, indicating hunger. However, this increase is just transient and often fades over time as your body adjusts to the fasting pattern. Some research suggests that intermittent fasting may help manage ghrelin levels, resulting in decreased hunger over time.

4. Leptin (The Satiety Hormone) regulates energy balance by signalling fullness to the brain.

Impact of fasting: Fasting increases leptin sensitivity, which means your body can better sense when it has ingested enough food, preventing overeating.

Cellular repair and autophagy.

Intermittent fasting induces autophagy, a normal biological mechanism in which the body degrades and recycles damaged cells. This process is critical to general health, ageing, and disease prevention.

What occurs during autophagy?

- Cellular cleanup: During a fast, cells begin to degrade old or malfunctioning components, such as broken proteins and organelles. This cleaning procedure is critical for preserving cellular health and function.
- Component recycling: The body recycles broken pieces and converts them into energy, which helps to revitalize cells.
- Disease prevention: Autophagy has been related to a lower risk of cancer, neurological illnesses, and cardiovascular disease. It protects your cells by eliminating poisons and dangerous chemicals.
- Autophagy typically begins after 16-24 hours of fasting, depending on the person. The longer you

fast, the more intense the autophagy process gets, resulting in better cell function and lifespan.

Effect on Insulin Sensitivity and Blood Sugar Regulation.

One of the most notable advantages of intermittent fasting is its potential to boost insulin sensitivity. Insulin sensitivity describes how well your cells react to insulin. Poor insulin sensitivity may lead to insulin resistance, which is a key risk factor for type 2 diabetes.

How fasting increases insulin sensitivity:

- Reduced insulin levels: Because insulin is a crucial factor in fat storage, fasting reduces insulin levels, which helps avoid excess fat buildup. This increased insulin sensitivity allows your body to absorb carbs more efficiently and maintain stable blood sugar levels.
- Reduced risk of type 2 diabetes. Intermittent fasting lowers insulin resistance, which reduces the chance of developing type 2 diabetes. Fasting has been demonstrated in studies to improve blood sugar control and minimize the requirement for insulin in those with pre-diabetes.

- Intermittent fasting may help diabetics and pre-diabetics manage their blood sugar levels. However, before beginning a fast, speak with a healthcare expert to verify that it is done safely.

Mental Clarity and Brain Health.

Fasting improves both your body and your intellect. During fasting, your body creates more brain-derived neurotrophic factor (BDNF), a protein that promotes brain health and functionality.

How Fasting Improves Brain Health:

- Increased BDNF: BDNF promotes neuronal development and survival, improves cognitive function, and protects against neurodegenerative illnesses such as Alzheimer's.
- Fasting has been demonstrated to improve neuroplasticity, or the brain's capacity to establish new connections and adapt to new knowledge. This leads to improved memory, learning, and mental clarity.
- Protection against brain ageing: Fasting may also protect the brain from oxidative stress and inflammation, which have been related to cognitive decline and neurodegenerative illnesses.

- Many individuals experience improved mental clarity and attention during fasting. This is related to the creation of ketones, which serve as a clean and efficient fuel supply for the brain.

Weight and Fat Loss.

The most well-known advantage of intermittent fasting is weight reduction, namely fat loss. Fasting promotes fat-burning and weight reduction by shortening the eating window and controlling insulin levels.

How fasting causes fat loss:

- Calorie reduction: By reducing your eating window, intermittent fasting naturally decreases your calorie intake, resulting in weight loss. Fasting may help manage hunger and portion sizes, so you may not need to watch calories.
- Increased fat burn: As we've seen, fasting causes your body's metabolism to shift from burning glucose to burning fat for energy, resulting in higher fat burning.
- Hormonal Benefits: As insulin levels drop during fasting, fat-burning hormones such as norepinephrine are produced, further promoting fat loss.

Intermittent fasting has been found in studies to significantly reduce body fat, especially in places such as the abdomen, where visceral fat (fat surrounding organs) is associated with increased health risks.

Longevity and ageing

Intermittent fasting has shown positive benefits to lifespan and ageing. Fasting may help delay the ageing process and lengthen life by improving systems such as autophagy and lowering inflammation.

How Fasting Affects Aging

- Improved mitochondrial function: Mitochondria are the cells' powerhouses and play an important role in ageing. Fasting enhances mitochondrial function, allowing cells to create energy more effectively and postponing age-related deterioration.
- Fasting reduces oxidative stress, which is linked to ageing and chronic illness. Fasting protects the body from free radical damage by boosting cellular repair.
- Increased longevity in animals: While human research is still being conducted, animal studies indicate that intermittent fasting may increase

longevity by enhancing metabolic health and lowering the risk of age-related illnesses.

Chapter 9:
Common Mistakes to Avoid While Fasting

Intermittent fasting may be a transforming practice, but like with any new lifestyle change, there is always the possibility of making errors along the way. Whether you're a novice or an experienced faster, avoiding common traps will help you make the most of your fasting experience. In this chapter, we will look at the most common errors individuals make during fasting and how to avoid them for long-term success.

Not staying hydrated.

One of the most frequent errors people make during fasting is failing to drink enough water. It is easy to forget to drink enough water during fasting, particularly over lengthy periods. Dehydration may induce tiredness, headaches, dizziness, and irritability, making fasting more difficult than necessary.

How to Avoid This Mistake:

- Drink plenty of water: Aim for at least 8 cups (64 ounces) of water every day, or more if you're active.

- Add electrolytes: If you're fasting for a long time, try adding a pinch of sea salt or drinking electrolyte water to restore lost minerals.
- Drink herbal tea or black coffee. These drinks may aid with hydration and are permitted during fasts as long as they do not include calories or sugar.

Overeating While Eating Windows

One of the most common hazards of intermittent fasting is overeating during the meal periods. Because you are fasting for a lengthy period, it may be tempting to eat huge quantities or consume harmful items after the fast is finished. Overeating might counteract the advantages of fasting, preventing weight reduction.

How to Avoid This Mistake:

- Focus on quality: Make sure your meals are nutritious and balanced, with lots of veggies, healthy fats, and lean meats.
- Mindful Eating: Eat carefully and pay attention to hunger signs. Stop eating when you are content, not full.
- Avoid bingeing. While it may seem like you need to "catch up" on food after fasting, bingeing may

cause stomach discomfort and upset your metabolism.

Not Consuming Enough Nutrients.

While it's crucial not to overeat, it's also critical not to undereat or overlook the nutritional value of your meals. Fasting shortens your eating window, and if you don't get enough nutrients, your body may struggle to operate properly, resulting in weariness, muscle loss, and other health difficulties.

How to Avoid This Mistake:

- Prioritize nutritious foods: Concentrate on entire foods such as leafy greens, lean meats, fish, eggs, nuts, seeds, and healthy fats like avocado and olive oil.
- Eat balanced meals. Each meal should have a combination of healthy fats, protein, and fibre to keep you satisfied and give you consistent energy throughout the day.
- Take vitamins if needed. If you discover that you are not receiving enough of specific vitamins or minerals (such as vitamin D or magnesium), you should consider adding a supplement to your regimen.

Fasting for too long or too often.

While fasting for longer periods might be beneficial, doing so too often or for too long can be harmful to your health. If you push yourself too hard, you may develop muscle loss, vitamin shortages, and other health problems. It's important to listen to your body and realize when it needs a break.

How to Avoid This Mistake:

- Begin with brief fasts: If you're new to fasting, start with 12- to 16-hour fasts and progressively expand your fasting window as your body adjusts.
- Take breaks. Do not feel the urge to fast every day. Having regular eating days or taking breaks from fasting might help you avoid fatigue and maintain a healthy balance.
- Pay heed to your body. If you feel lightheaded, tired, or weak, it might be because you're fasting for too long or too often. Listen to your body and make adjustments to your fasting schedule as needed.

Skipping Meals Following the Fast

Some individuals make the mistake of missing meals after breaking their fast, thinking it would help them lose more weight. However, missing meals might upset your metabolism, resulting in overeating later in the day. Your body needs fuel to operate correctly, particularly after a fast.

How to Avoid This Mistake:

- Eat a balanced meal. After breaking your fast, eat a well-balanced meal rich in healthy fats, protein, and fibre to restore your body's energy reserves and promote muscle recovery.
- Do not miss breakfast. If you're following a daily intermittent fasting regimen, don't miss breakfast or your first meal after the fast. Skipping meals might lead to overeating later in the day, slowing your progress.
- Small meals to begin: If you're new to fasting, it's OK to start with a smaller meal following your fast and gradually increase as your body adjusts to fasting.

Not getting enough sleep.

Sleep is a crucial component of any healthy lifestyle, yet fasting may make it difficult to obtain enough sleep if not done correctly. Sleep deprivation may raise hunger hormones, weaken willpower, and result in bad eating decisions. It may also have a detrimental impact on your metabolism and weight reduction objectives.

How to Avoid This Mistake:

- Prioritize sleep. Aim for 7-9 hours of good sleep every night. Sleep is essential for muscle repair, development, and hormone balance.
- Avoid taking caffeine late in the day. If you're fasting and ingesting coffee, be cautious of when you consume it. Avoid coffee at least 6 hours before bedtime to avoid disrupting your sleep.
- Create a sleep-friendly atmosphere. Make your bedroom dark, quiet, and cold to encourage good sleep.

Ignoring the need for physical activity.

It's crucial to be physically active when fasting to retain muscle mass, increase metabolism, and boost fat-burning. Some individuals feel that fasting alone will result in weight reduction, but physical activity is an important part of reaching your objectives.

How to Avoid This Mistake:

- Incorporate regular exercise. Aim for at least 3-4 days of physical activity each week, with a variety of cardio, weight training, and flexibility activities.
- Listen to your body: If you're fasting and feeling exhausted, reduce the intensity of your exercises, but don't miss them.
- Focus on strength training: Incorporate weight training to help you maintain muscle mass while shedding fat. Muscle improves metabolism and promotes long-term fat reduction.

Not being patient

Intermittent fasting produces results over time, and impatience may lead to dissatisfaction. Some individuals quit fasting early because they do not notice quick effects, yet perseverance is the key to success.

How to Avoid This Mistake:

- Trust the process. Significant weight and body composition changes might take weeks if not months. Stay dedicated and concentrate on long-term outcomes.

- Track your progress: Keep track of your progress by recording your weight, body fat percentage, energy levels, and mental state. Progress is not always linear, but constant work yields results over time.
- Be flexible: If one fasting schedule or strategy isn't working for you, don't be scared to try something else. The trick is to determine what works best for your body.

Fasting Without a Clear Goal.

Fasting without a specific objective in mind might seem aimless and disheartening. Having defined, quantifiable objectives can help you remain motivated and guarantee that your efforts produce the required results.

How to Avoid This Mistake:

- Set clear objectives. Set precise, actionable objectives to keep you motivated, such as decreasing weight, increasing energy, or lowering inflammation.
- Measure your progress: Track your progress with measurements, images, or how you feel physically

and psychologically. This will allow you to remain on target and change your strategy as needed.

Chapter 10:

Factors to Consider When Choosing a Fasting Schedule

When choosing a fasting schedule, consider your demands and lifestyle. Here are some elements to consider while developing your unique fasting plan:

1. Your goals:

Are you fasting mainly to lose weight, increase energy, or enhance general health? For weight reduction, a plan like 16/8 or 5:2 may be useful, although more sophisticated schedules like Eat-Stop-Eat may provide more drastic outcomes.

2. Your everyday Routine:

Do you have a set job schedule, family obligations, or other everyday activities? Choose a fasting approach that compliments your daily schedule and helps you manage your time wisely.

3. Your Hunger Level:

Some individuals naturally have a larger appetite in the morning, whilst others may feel hungry at night.

Choose a timetable that corresponds to your body's normal hunger cycles, so you don't have to resist its signals.

4. Physical activity level:

If you exercise often, try using a fasting strategy that offers adequate energy for your exercises, such as the 16/8 approach, which allows you to eat after your workout. For more rigorous fasting regimens, such as OMAD or Eat-Stop-Eat, you may want to plan your meals around your exercises to maximize performance.

5. Your health status:

If you have any medical concerns (such as diabetes, thyroid disorders, or heart disease), you should contact a healthcare expert before beginning any fasting regimen. Certain conditions need more careful or modified fasting procedures.

How to Begin Your Fasting Plan

Once you've decided on a fasting strategy that meets your requirements, it's time to put it into action. Here's a step-by-step tutorial to get you started:

- **Step 1: Select your fasting schedule.**

Choose a fasting schedule that fits your lifestyle. If you're a newbie, start with a modest approach like 16/8 and move to more advanced ways as you gain confidence in fasting.

- **Step 2: Set a start date.**

Choose a date to start your fasting adventure. It's best to start at the beginning of the week to establish a routine, but the time is ultimately up to you.

- **Step 3: Prepare your meals.**

Plan your meals ahead of time to ensure that they are nutritious and pleasant. Include a mix of healthy fats, proteins, and fibre-rich carbs to keep you satisfied throughout mealtimes.

- **Step 4: Start Slowly**

If you're new to fasting, begin with a shorter fasting period (e.g., 12 hours) and gradually increase it as your body adapts. Do not feel compelled to begin lengthier fasts immediately.

- **Step 5: Monitor your progress.**

Track your success by keeping track of your meal times, energy levels, mood, and any physical changes, such as weight or body measurements. Keeping note of your experiences will allow you to determine what works best for you.

- **Step 6: Adjust as needed.**

Listen to your body. If you feel lightheaded, exhausted, or extremely hungry, your fasting schedule may need to be adjusted. Consider reducing your fasting period or adjusting your eating window to meet your demands.

Sample Fasting Schedules

To get you started, here are some examples of varied fasting schedules:

1. 16/8 Method (Time-Restricted Eating):

- Eating hours: 12 PM - 8 PM.
- Fasting Hours: 8 PM - 12 PM (following day).
- Example meals:
- Noon: Grilled chicken salad with olive oil dressing.
- 3 p.m.: Greek yoghurt with berries and almonds
- 7 p.m.: Salmon with roasted veggies.

2. The 5:2 method (alternate-day fasting)

- Eating days: Monday, Wednesday, Friday, Saturday, and Sunday (regular eating).
- Fasting Days: Tuesday, Thursday (500-600 calories)
- Example Meals for Fasting Days:
- Meal One: Broth-based vegetable soup
- Meal 2: Small salad with cooked eggs and olive oil.

3. The OMAD Method (One Meal a Day):

- Eating Hours: 1 PM - 2 PM.
- Fasting Hours: 2 PM - 1 PM (following day).
- Example Meal: 1 PM: Grilled steak with steamed broccoli, quinoa, and avocado.

Chapter 11:

Overcoming Common Challenges While Fasting

While intermittent fasting has numerous advantages, it is not without drawbacks. From coping with hunger sensations to handling social settings, the path may not always be easy. However, recognizing the major challenges that individuals experience and how to overcome them will help you stay motivated and make fasting a long-term lifestyle choice.

1. Hunger and cravings.

Hunger is one of the most difficult obstacles when beginning intermittent fasting, particularly in the early stages. Cravings for sweet or salty meals may also lead you to break your fast early. These sentiments are normal, and there are ways to handle them.

How to solve the challenge:
- Stay hydrated. Thirst may sometimes be mistaken for hunger. Drink lots of water throughout the day, and try drinking herbal teas to satisfy cravings.

- Consume fibre-rich meals: During your eating windows, choose high-fibre meals like vegetables, whole grains, and legumes to keep you feeling filled for longer.
- Distract yourself. Engage in an activity that gets your attention off eating, such as a hobby, a stroll, or a phone call with a friend.
- Gradual adaptation: If you're new to fasting, start with shorter fasting periods and gradually extend them as your body adjusts to the fasting practice.

2. Low energy levels.

When individuals initially start fasting, they may feel fatigued or have low energy levels. This may happen when your body adapts to using fat for energy rather than carbs. While this is usually only transitory, there are techniques to control it and keep your energy levels consistent.

How to solve the challenge:

- Ensure optimal nutrition: During eating periods, emphasize nutrient-dense meals with a balanced mix of healthy fats, protein, and fibre. These will help you maintain your blood sugar levels and stay energetic.

- Get enough rest: Sleep is essential for keeping energy levels stable. Aim for 7-9 hours of sleep every night to help your body recuperate and maintain high energy levels.
- Exercise at the appropriate time: If you are feeling tired, consider exercising during your meal window rather than when fasting. This will guarantee that you have adequate energy for your exercise.
- Be patient: As your body adjusts to fasting, the energy dips will diminish. Allow your body time to acclimate to the new regimen.

3. Social Situations & Dining Out

Social gatherings and meals with friends and family may be difficult to manage while fasting. Attending food-focused gatherings may make it tough to keep to your fasting strategy, particularly if others are eating around you.

How to solve the challenge:
- Plan. If you know you'll be attending a social event or dining out during your eating window, prepare your meals ahead of time. This may help you remain on target and prevent overeating.

- Bring your meal: If you're attending an event where you won't have many alternatives, consider bringing your food. This will guarantee that you eat something nutritious and consistent with your fasting objectives.
- Be aware and not rigid: If you need to break your fast or change your eating schedule for a particular event, don't feel bad. One meal will not undo your progress. The idea is to get back on track as quickly as possible.
- Set boundaries: If you're fasting at a social function, don't be afraid to calmly explain why. Most people will appreciate your decision, which will help alleviate any pressure to eat.

4. Plateaus and Slow Progress

As you proceed with intermittent fasting, you may reach a plateau when weight reduction or other health advantages seem to stop. This might be disappointing, particularly if you saw fast effects at first. However, plateaus are common and may be surmounted.

How to solve the challenge:

- Evaluate your approach: If you've been fasting for a while and haven't noticed any results, it may be time to reconsider your fasting schedule or eating habits. You may need to change your meal schedule, calorie consumption, or exercise program.

- Track your progress: Instead of focusing simply on weight, look for other signals of change, such as more energy, improved mood, better sleep, or less inflammation. These indicators may suggest success even if the scale does not move.
- Change up your routine: Our bodies can adapt to the same pattern. To shock your system and break through the plateau, experiment with alternative fasting patterns or increase the intensity of your exercises.

5. Emotional Eating & Stress

Emotional eating is another prevalent issue while fasting. Stress, worry, or boredom may all induce a want to eat outside of your fasting window. This emotional attachment to food may be a significant obstacle to success.

How to solve the challenge:

- Address the emotional triggers: Identify the emotions or events that trigger emotional eating.

Keep a diary to chronicle your emotions and eating habits, which can help you identify better methods to deal with stress.
- Discover alternate coping techniques. Instead of turning to food when you're worried, consider deep breathing techniques, yoga, meditation, or a soothing stroll.
- Practice mindfulness. When eating during your windows, remember to be present and aware. Pay attention to your hunger and fullness indicators, and only eat when you're hungry. Mindful eating may help you stop the pattern of emotional eating.

6. Cravings for sweets or junk foods

Many individuals have strong desires for sweet or processed meals, particularly during fasting. These cravings may be particularly powerful in the early stages when your body is accustomed to using fat for fuel rather than sugar.

How to solve the challenge:
- Avoid trigger foods: Keeping sweets or junk food accessible might make it difficult to resist

temptation. Stock your kitchen with healthful foods like fruits, almonds, and dark chocolate.
- Choose healthier alternatives: If you want something sweet, try natural sweeteners like stevia or monk fruit, or eat a piece of fruit. These solutions might satisfy your sweet desires without interrupting your fast.
- Keep busy: Distracting yourself with an activity or interest might help you avoid cravings. To keep yourself engaged during these cravings, do something you like, such as reading, crocheting, or working out.

7. Getting Used to Long-Term Fasting

The first few weeks of fasting may be tough, but after your body adapts, fasting may become second nature. However, maintaining consistency and motivation over time might be difficult, particularly if you don't notice quick benefits or encounter setbacks.

How to solve the challenge:

- Track your development regularly. As previously said, monitoring progress with images, measurements, and non-scale successes will help you stay motivated. Celebrate minor victories to keep motivated.

- Create a routine. Create a regular fasting schedule that works with your lifestyle. Consistency is essential for making fasting a sustainable discipline. Fasting will become a natural part of your everyday routine.
- Maintain flexibility: Life will always have highs and lows. If you miss a fasting window or need to change your practice, don't be too harsh on yourself. Maintain flexibility and keep your long-term objectives in mind.

Conclusion:
Your New Lifestyle – Making Fasting a Lifelong Habit

Congratulations on making it this far! You've learned about the science of intermittent fasting, various fasting regimens, the advantages it may provide, and how to tailor your fasting experience. Now is the moment to make intermittent fasting a permanent part of your lifestyle—a lifetime practice that can improve your health and quality of life.

Intermittent fasting is neither a temporary diet nor a quick remedy. It's a strong tool that can help you regain your health, increase your energy, and enhance your general well-being. Whether you want to lose weight, increase your mental clarity, or improve your general health, intermittent fasting is a versatile and successful technique that can be tailored to your specific goals. More significantly, fasting is about making long-term changes. Adopting intermittent fasting as a lifestyle prepares you for a future full of vitality, energy, and long-term health advantages. Here's how to make fasting a lifetime habit.

The Road Ahead: Adopting Fasting as a Lifelong Habit

Intermittent fasting is more than simply a diet or fad. It is a long-term lifestyle modification that may lead to improved health, longevity, and well-being. Fasting regularly may help you become a healthier, happier version of yourself.

Remember that the intermittent fasting path is unique to each individual. There will be highs and lows, but if you stick to your objectives, stay flexible, and listen to your body, you will achieve long-term success.
Here's to your new healthy, lively, and energy-filled lifestyle. May intermittent fasting be the key to realizing your greatest potential and changing your life.
Thank you for reading!

Thank you for selecting Fast to Fit: The Ultimate Intermittent Fasting Handbook. We hope this book has given you the information and encouragement you need to adopt intermittent fasting and make it a lifetime habit. Your health transformation begins now—take the first step and enjoy the trip ahead!

Bonus Section: Your Ultimate Guide to Fasting Success

To conclude your intermittent fasting adventure, we've created a Bonus Section with some of the most commonly asked questions, an example 7-day intermittent fasting schedule, and meal prep suggestions for your eating windows. These materials can help you remain on track and get the most out of your fasting lifestyle.

Sample 7-Day Intermittent Fasting Plan

This 7-day sample plan follows the 16:8 fasting method, where you fast for 16 hours and eat within an 8-hour window. You can adjust the eating times based on your schedule.

Day 1 (Monday)

- **Fasting window**: 8:00 PM – 12:00 PM
- **Eating window**: 12:00 PM – 8:00 PM
- **Meals**:
    - **Lunch**: Grilled chicken salad with avocado, olive oil, and mixed greens
    - **Snack**: Handful of almonds
    - **Dinner**: Baked salmon with roasted Brussels sprouts and quinoa

Day 2 (Tuesday)

- **Fasting window**: 7:00 PM – 11:00 AM
- **Eating window**: 11:00 AM – 7:00 PM
- **Meals**:
    - **Lunch**: Turkey lettuce wraps with hummus, cucumber, and bell peppers
    - **Snack**: Greek yoghurt with chia seeds
    - **Dinner**: Stir-fried tofu with vegetables and cauliflower rice

Day 3 (Wednesday)

- **Fasting window**: 6:00 PM – 10:00 AM
- **Eating window**: 10:00 AM – 6:00 PM
- **Meals**:
    - **Lunch**: Scrambled eggs with spinach and avocado
    - **Snack**: Sliced apple with almond butter
    - **Dinner**: Grilled shrimp with a side of roasted sweet potatoes and steamed broccoli

Day 4 (Thursday)

- **Fasting window**: 8:00 PM – 12:00 PM
- **Eating window**: 12:00 PM – 8:00 PM
- **Meals**:

- **Lunch**: Chicken and vegetable stir-fry with olive oil and soy sauce
- **Snack**: Celery with cream cheese
- **Dinner**: Grass-fed beef burger with a side of mixed green salad and avocado

Day 5 (Friday)

- **Fasting window**: 7:00 PM – 11:00 AM
- **Eating window**: 11:00 AM – 7:00 PM
- **Meals**:
  - **Lunch**: Tuna salad with mixed greens, olive oil, and lemon dressing
  - **Snack**: Hard-boiled eggs
  - **Dinner**: Grilled chicken thighs with zucchini noodles and pesto

Day 6 (Saturday)

- **Fasting window**: 9:00 PM – 1:00 PM
- **Eating window**: 1:00 PM – 9:00 PM
- **Meals**:
  - **Lunch**: Cobb salad with grilled chicken, avocado, hard-boiled eggs, and ranch dressing
  - **Snack**: Trail mix (nuts and dried fruit)

- **Dinner**: Baked cod with roasted carrots and wild rice

Day 7 (Sunday)

- **Fasting window**: 8:00 PM – 12:00 PM
- **Eating window**: 12:00 PM – 8:00 PM
- **Meals**:
    - **Lunch**: Grilled salmon with asparagus and quinoa
    - **Snack**: Sliced cucumber with guacamole
    - **Dinner**: Roasted chicken with steamed green beans and mashed cauliflower

Meal Prep Ideas for Eating Windows

To make the most of your eating window, meal prepping is an excellent way to save time, stay on track, and ensure that you have healthy meals ready to go. Here are some meal prep ideas for your fasting journey:

- **Grilled chicken breasts**: Grill a batch of chicken breasts at the start of the week and use them in salads, wraps, or stir-fries.
- **Chopped vegetables**: Prepare a variety of vegetables (broccoli, cauliflower, bell peppers, zucchini) for quick stir-fries or to steam as sides.
- **Hard-boiled eggs**: A great high-protein snack that can be prepared in advance and eaten throughout the week.
- **Overnight oats**: Prepare single-serving jars of overnight oats for a quick and healthy breakfast.
- **Quinoa or brown rice**: Cook a large batch of quinoa or brown rice to use as a base for meals throughout the week.
- **Roasted vegetables**: Roast vegetables such as sweet potatoes, carrots, or Brussels sprouts to pair with proteins.

- **Homemade salads**: Prepare a few mason jar salads with leafy greens, toppings, and dressing on the side for a quick, grab-and-go meal.

1.

Made in the USA
Columbia, SC
03 January 2025